I0151612

Testimonials

Obsessive-Compulsive Disorder (O. C. D.) is a genuine mental health condition that profoundly impacted my brother's life from a young age. As a caring family, we were unaware of this disorder until he reached a point of acknowledging its presence in his early adulthood.

As I delved into his narrative, it was disheartening to learn about the challenges he faced during his adult years, reflecting on potential indicators that the disorder might have surfaced in his elementary school days. Witnessing the reemergence of OCD symptoms when he was accidentally struck in the face by a Coca-Cola bottle cap heightened our concern, leading us to fervently pray for the day he would find the necessary support.

Reading through his journey, I found solace in the realization that his wife, Patty, and their children played a pivotal role in providing the love and support that empowered my brother to navigate and manage his daily life. His story is a testament to resilience and triumph, as he not only acknowledged his struggle with OCD, but also took control, enabling himself to build a fulfilling family life and retire in a profession he cherished.

It is my hope that his story will resonate with others, reassuring them that they are not alone and that assistance is available.

-Mike Ramirez

Don't Panic was a thought-provoking read. I couldn't put it down.

It's amazing to see the progress and transformation that's possible in the mental health arena. I recommend this book to anyone who experiences —or knows someone who experiences— mental health challenges.

This book will provide a glimpse of hope!

-Autumn Medina

Don't Panic is a very good and informative book that I was able to relate to. I also suffered from anxiety and stress in my middle age and was tormented with the same evil unexplainable feelings.

I strongly recommend this book to all readers that may be suffering from unknown feelings of fear, disorientation, and confusion.

-Gilbert Ramirez

Adrian has been an inspiration to me because I have seen the struggles he has gone through over the years with his OCD as much as the progress he is making in coping with this condition. Just him knowing and acknowledging that he has a problem shows me how strong of a person he is.

-Frank Medina

Don't PANIC

MY LIFE STORY

Adrian Ramirez

Don't Panic

My Life Story

Halo
PUBLISHING
INTERNATIONAL

Copyright © 2024 Adrian Ramirez, All rights reserved.

No part of this publication may be reproduced, stored in a retrieval system or transmitted in any form or by any means, electronic, mechanical, photocopying, recording or otherwise, without prior permission of Halo Publishing International.

The views and opinions expressed in this book are those of the author and do not necessarily reflect the official policy or position of Halo Publishing International. Any content provided by our authors are of their opinion and are not intended to malign any religion, ethnic group, club, organization, company, individual or anyone or anything.

For permission requests, write to the publisher, addressed "Attention: Permissions Coordinator," at the address below.

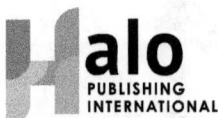

Halo
PUBLISHING
INTERNATIONAL

Halo Publishing International
7550 WIH-10 #800, PMB 2069,
San Antonio, TX 78229

First Edition, April 2024
ISBN: 978-1-63765-594-8
Library of Congress Control Number: 2024906567

The information contained within this book is strictly for informational purposes. Unless otherwise indicated, all the names, characters, businesses, places, events and incidents in this book are either the product of the author's imagination or used in a fictitious manner. Any resemblance to actual persons, living or dead, or actual events is purely coincidental.

Halo Publishing International is a self-publishing company that publishes adult fiction and non-fiction, children's literature, self-help, spiritual, and faith-based books. We continually strive to help authors reach their publishing goals and provide many different services that help them do so. We do not publish books that are deemed to be politically, religiously, or socially disrespectful, or books that are sexually provocative, including erotica. Halo reserves the right to refuse publication of any manuscript if it is deemed not to be in line with our principles. Do you have a book idea you would like us to consider publishing? Please visit www.halopublishing.com for more information.

Dedicated to:

Manijeh and Dr. Habib Nathan, MD Psychiatry, and his staff of counselors;

Dr. Mark Drogin, MD Psychiatry;

Rebecca Medina, beloved sister-in-law;

My family, for all of their love and support throughout the years.

Contents

Introduction

This book will take you into my brain, which has a biological condition that affects the way I can think in an unimaginable and unrealistic sense. The condition I am referring to is known as Obsessive-Compulsive Disorder (O.C.D.). With this disorder come symptoms that include anxiety and panic attacks, which can cripple you mentally. It doesn't discriminate by race, sex, gender or age.

Growing up I had no idea there was even a name for the way my mind controlled me, the way it lied to me, the way my own being and soul would be taken from me. I merely thought I had a nervous condition that someday I would grow out of.

I grew up living the darkest moments of horror within my own self. Only those of us who suffer with these conditions will ever know what it is like to live having to make a way through a dark cloud of shame, hurt, fear, and sadness. With the use of medication and therapy I have been able to walk through that dark and scary cloud and can now see what life should be like without having to live each day in horror within my own self.

I was blessed to be diagnosed at an age that was very crucial in my life; to find out it is a rare condition, something I have no control of and to know that it is not me going crazy but simply a genetic factor that is flowing within my blood stream. As those who are genetically inclined to have high blood pressure or diabetes, I inherited what I consider to be the demon's worst mental condition. One that makes you think of terrible things within a millisecond and can last for hours at times, even days. For it to seem so real as if watching a horrific movie clip that keeps playing over and over in the mind, making one go into crying antics of fear and confusion.

I wrote this book to let others in the world know that there is a cure, and though it will never go away completely, it can be treated and manageable to live with. It may take a few days or months but, like a baby learns to walk, we too must take those baby steps to get back to where we once were in our lives. We can't let this mental beast manipulate us to the point that we lose all we have.

My College Years

It was 1981 and I was going to San Antonio College in San Antonio, Texas. This college was best known as a continuation of our high school due to the amount of former class-mates that attended. I guess you could say that during that time it was looked down on as a Junior College, being that those like me who didn't excel in high school would go there to start off a college education. A little embarrassing, I could say, being that my girlfriend Patty was attending St. Mary's University, majoring in Business. I always felt I was not up to her caliber, but she loved me then, now, and was and has always been my rock. During this time, I had a part time job at a major department store and worked in the hardware section.

Well, it was almost spring-time and I went to Patty's house to pick her up after work one day. It was a Friday night and the movies was the place to go. As we left her home, Patty looked at me in a way I had never been seen before. She informed me that she thought she might be pregnant. My heart began to beat heavy and my hands started to sweat. I couldn't believe what she was telling me. There was no way. Well, yes, there was, because we had had sex, but my mind was saying no because we both had to finish college and her parents had very high expectations of her.

As a few months went by, it was true, Patty was pregnant and it was time for me to make a major decision. The fear of telling my parents was not as bad as the fear of telling my older brother Mike, who constantly was on about me finishing college. I could hear him already, "I told you, whatever you do, make sure Patty does not get pregnant". For days I tossed and turned in bed at night, wondering how I was going to break the news to my parents, brothers and sisters.

One morning I finally developed the courage and told my mother. I had thought long and hard about it and decided I had to be a real father, I had to take on the responsibility. My child would not grow up without a father in his life.

I later went and spoke with Patty's parents, with great embarrassment of course. Her brother Frank was my hero and spoke up for me, he explained that I was not a bad guy and that I was willing to take on the responsibility.

Patty had already told him that she was going to finish college and I would find a full-time job.

We agreed to get married as soon as possible. The plans were to have a garden wedding in the backyard of her sister Dolores' residence. She had the beautiful yard with the nice trees, etc. Patty's nephew, Michael, would be the DJ with some home-equipment he had in his room. I can tell you that, until this day, it is all a haze to me. All that time I was in that cloud and I had no idea what was going on. However, for some reason I was feeling good considering I was now getting married, having a child; soon to be a husband and father. Little did I know how dark that cloud hovering over me was about to get.

While the arrangements were being made for the wedding, Patty and I went to search for and see some inexpensive apartments. The most affordable apartment we could find was an efficiency two-bedroom. With no furniture or credit to buy furniture, we settled for hand me downs from family and whatever little I had and she had from home. At the same time, I was offered a full-time position at the department store.

The wedding came and so did the rain. Our plans for a garden wedding flooded away in thunderstorms. Her parents were able to find a small hall and the celebration went on as planned. We spent our honeymoon in our small apartment, sleeping on a twin-size bed.

The Dark Cloud
Returns

On January 24th, 1981, my son Bryan was born. I was so excited about becoming a father. We had our child at the Robert B. Green Hospital known for low-income-patients. As the nursing staff prepared Patty for delivery, I was asked if I could go and pick up an order of Chinese food for the doctor. By the time I returned, Patty was in the delivery room. I was allowed to enter to witness the birth of our first child. My little boy arrived, a full head of dark black hair and rosy cheeks. Wow, I was now a dad.

The months prior, my mind had been going and going since the day Patty had informed me that she was pregnant. I don't think anything else was on my mind. I was on overdrive getting married, a full-time job now, an apartment, and a baby born. It would soon be time to take our baby home to our little apartment, one small living area combined with the dining and kitchen and two small bedrooms and a bath down a small hallway. Simply put, it could be referred to as a matchbox.

Our son Bryan was such a cute little baby and I was very happy, though our finances were taking a toll on me already. I would not, however, let that get in the way of the love I had for my son. He laid there in his room, peaceful as a little angel in his crib with the everyday crying and hunger as any other baby. I shared the time with Patty and we learned very fast what it was like to be parents.

One Friday evening my brother Mike called to let us know that he and my sister-in-law, Cathy, were coming over to see the baby. Once they arrived, Mike and I went to the grocery store to buy some snacks, including a soda. We returned to the apartment and Patty was with Cathy and our son in the living area.

I went to the kitchen and began to serve drinks. As I attempted to remove the cap off of the 48 oz. soda bottle for the drinks, POW, the cap flew off and it struck me in the eye. I was hit so hard that I fainted in the bathroom. I don't know if it was due to the hit or the impression of looking at my face and eye. My eye was bleeding and I was blind. A rumbling fear swept through my body as I began to shake.

Mike took me to the hospital. I began to lose my breath and became very nervous. The doctor asked me to place my hand over my good eye and look at a board with alphabets. The shock and fear became stronger and stronger when I realized that I could not see. I was told that my eyeball had been damaged by the metal of the soda bottle cap. A patch was placed on my eye and I was told to go and see an eye specialist the following day.

I made it back home and at one point I began to hyperventilate. Patty asked, "What is wrong with you?" She kept telling me not to worry, that I was going to be alright. I felt like a child in a man's body wanting to hear those words from his mommy. My mind would not accept what she was saying and I began to cry uncontrollably, I was in fear of losing my eyesight.

The next day I had a terrible headache and a cloud of fear came over my soul. I was very depressed and anxious, I had so much anxiety that I could not hold on to my son Bryan. I was now in that dark cloud again. The cloud of fear, torment, frustration, anger, the unknown.

"Oh nooooo," I told Patty, "I am just realizing something. This is the way I would feel when I was a kid in elementary school. It's back." "No way it's back!", she had no idea what I was talking about.

Days went by and I could not shake the feeling of fear. Telling myself and Patty, "It must just be the immediate shock that got to me, the fact that I may lose my eyesight." By this time I now had some vision and was told by the specialist that I was going to be okay. But, that feeling? That ugly, possessed feeling, I still had it? Why?

It was now a Monday morning and Patty had to go to the University for a major exam. I forced myself to help her get Bryan ready for daycare. I was still recovering from my injury, staying at home, missing work and not getting paid. As she left, I sat down and began to watch a movie that was showing which contained violence. All of a sudden, for some unknown reason, I could not watch it anymore. The movie made me feel strange inside, the fear in me grew every time a violent scene showed. The walls and rooms in the apartment appeared to be coming down on me. I was floating in that dark cloud. My heart raced, my body was sweating, my stomach ached and I felt light headed. I was out of control in my own self.

I would walk back and forth in the small apartment, wondering what was going on with me, grabbing my head as I sat on the couch. A feeling of despair and horror was once again back in my life. I was embarrassed, to say the least, but more so very scared, like a child left in a store looking for their parent. I could not take it anymore so I got dressed and went to my parents to speak with my mother about the way I felt, I craved the comfort of her, who I knew was home alone. Dad was at work. I remembered my mother once saying that when a person gets scared you must give them some sugar for the immediate shock. She would say it must be done so they don't get "El Susto", which in Spanish means "The Fear".

As I got dressed, I trembled. Here I was, 19 years of age and wanting to go be with Mommy. It must be a child instinct because I felt like a baby at the time.

As I entered her home I sat on the dining room chair. My mom looked at me and said, "What's wrong with you, son, your eyes are very dark". I then began to sob uncontrollably, saying, "Mom, Mom, oh please, Mom, help me, it's back. It's back. Mom."

"What is it, son?" she replied. "That feeling I used to get when I was a kid, remember when I didn't want to go to school?"

She wrapped her arms around me and held on tight as I cried and cried. She too began to weep, saying, "*Ay, Mijo.*" Which in Spanish means "Oh, my son". My mom did speak English, but spoke her native language at times.

I explained to my mother that I had not slept well for days. My mother told me to lay down on the sofa and relax as she made me a herbal tea that would calm my nerves. I don't know if it was a psychological game she was playing with me or not, but it worked. I drank that tea and as I laid my head down on the sofa I fell asleep like my newborn son.

I later awoke and went back to the apartment. Thanking my mother before I left, I could see she was still worried as she blessed me on the way out the door.

Patty would later arrive with our son Bryan and I went downstairs to the parking lot of the apartment complex to help her with our son and her books from school. "How you feeling, hun?" she said. I replied with "Oh, much better, sweetie."

I knew I was not feeling one hundred percent better, but managed to tell her that so that she would not worry. She had enough on her mind with our new born son and her college studies. I was just happy and felt some comfort knowing she was home and I had someone to talk to.

Later that evening, as the sun began to settle, that feeling of anxiety and fear started to creep up on me again. Patty could see that I was not doing well.

"What's wrong?" Patty asked. "Oh nothing, why?" She knew me too well. I told her that I was going to be okay and that I had gone to see my mother and she had this great tea to drink. I could see she was starting to get concerned. Patty was upset that I had gone to see my mother, she was afraid that now my mother would be worried about me. I reassured her that my mother was fine.

I was not telling her the truth, in case I needed to go back.

The O. C. D. Attack

A few weeks had gone by. I was walking around like an old frail man, unshaven, wrinkled clothes, and a feeling of hopelessness. What is it? Why has it come back? Is God punishing me for something I did wrong? That was it. I should have never asked myself that question about God. It took its toll on my spirit and kicked my OCD into motion.

Now, growing up I did not battle with any obsessive-compulsive disorders that I can remember. I did, though, suffer from severe anxiety and panic attacks. But now my battle with the OCD monster had come to play.

I asked God if He was mad about that time I got into a fight with that kid in high school? Oh no, did he die? Oh noooooooooo, am I going to go to prison for murder? Oh noooooo. Oh noooooo. Or is it about that girl I kissed in high school? Did she have my baby? Did we have sex? Did I do something I was not supposed to do? Oh noooooooooo. Nooooooooooo... Why Lord? Why? Why am I thinking these things? Are they real?

Maybe it is true. Maybe I did do something that I don't remember doing. How now do I tell

Patty what I am thinking? Patty walked by and saw me crying on the sofa. "Now what, Adrian? You were doing fine earlier." "Patty, I am getting some weird thoughts. I am thinking I may have hurt someone or even killed them." Patty, by this time, began to get emotional and worried. She was trying to diagnose my problem but did not know the answer. Things started to escalate.

I began to ask Patty not to leave me alone, I didn't want to be home alone. She had no choice but to leave for school. The nights were comfortable once I fell asleep next to her, but I dreaded the morning as I did in my days as a young kid. I was in the apartment alone and desperate, praying and praying to God. This feeling felt evil, the thoughts were evil. I decided to go and see a Priest. Perhaps this feeling I had was an evil spirit that had entered my body. I was so desperate that I went right up to the Catholic Church we used to attend and knocked on the Priest's residency building.

I asked to speak to the Priest. I was like a drug addict wanting some dope, I needed a fix and I needed it now. The Priest spoke to me and I remember him telling me that time had caught up to me, I was young and had been hit with a lot of different things. I was now married with a child, out of work due to my injury, which made us financially strapped, etc.; too many logs in the fire as the old saying goes. He blessed me and prayed over my soul. Did it help? No. By the time I got back to our apartment I was just as bad.

Patty and I would eventually sit down to analyze my condition. Perhaps it was the apartment, it was too small and I didn't have anywhere to go. The only thing I could do was step out on the balcony which looked over the parking lot. It was decided that we would move to a house for rent. Maybe being in a house, and a change of scenery, would help me.

Within time, Patty could no longer take it. We moved into the house and the devil was still in me. I say the devil because the intrusive thoughts that flooded my mind were as if Satan was talking to me, putting bad thoughts in my head over and over again. By now I was also taking trips to the Emergency Room to be examined. The fear of going crazy was driving me insane. My chest was tight, my stomach ached, my mouth had a taste of rust, a fever like heat and a floating sensation as if my soul had left my body. Over and over the doctor would say there was nothing wrong.

The only prescription I got was advice not to allow life get to me. I kept hearing the same thing over and over. "Maybe you just have too much on your mind."

Patty was suffering along with me and at one point told my mother-in-law about my condition. My mother-in-law knew of a Witch Doctor, known to many Hispanics of Mexican descent as a *Curandera*. By now I was willing to try anything to take away these thoughts, anxiety, panic and this abnormal feeling.

We went to this *Curandera*. These *curanderas* normally live in dark areas of town. I was not a big believer in them, however, if she could perform a miracle, I would take it. As we entered the residence I could see garlic hanging on the walls, religious candles burning and perceived a smell of moth balls. I was introduced to this elderly lady who walked up to me. She was about 5'1" tall, dark complexion with gray stringy hair. She began to say things over me as I stood there. She told me not to be afraid and that I had to believe in her, she seemed to sense something over me and said that something I saw had scared me and taken over my spirit. She reached over to a small wooden table and placed her wrinkled hand into a bowl, she grabbed a small salt rock and began to rub it all over my head. As she was doing this, prayed and said things in her own words. The object of this procedure was to rub the rock on me and then place it on a steel hot plate she had warming up. The plate, called a *comal*, a utensil for making tortillas, was waiting for the rock. On this plate there was a small gap which is used for grabbing with a tool to place it in hot water. Once the *Curandera* was done, she placed the small salt rock on this hot plate. The salt rock was to melt into an image of what it was that was attacking my spirit.

Once again, my luck would keep going bad. The salt rock began to melt and fell into the small gap of the hot plate and till this day I will never know what the image would have been. Whatever it is she did, it did not help either.

One day as I sat around moping, my hair in a mess, unshaven and feeling sick. Yes, I say sick because it feels like a stomach virus with only the aching stomach and chills. I was depressed and not wanting to do anything. Patty demanded that I get up, take a shower, shave and that we get out and go somewhere. She didn't care where, she just wanted to get out of the house because now she was starting to get depressed.

She noticed that every time I was at home I would start to get worse. I can say that she was the first therapist I had and she never gave up on me. She seemed to know what I needed, I needed to keep my mind active, not to allow myself to relax and in get into a state of mind conducive to dwelling on my intrusive thoughts.

As the symptoms would creep up on me she would give me something to do whether it was to go to the store or work on the yard. I was not to stay idle by no means. Through her therapy session, the symptoms eventually subsided like flood waters and I was back on track. Within a few weeks I went to work and eventually found a new job and we later bought a house.

The Return
of the Monster

It had now been seven years with no OCD symptoms, no intrusive thoughts, panic attacks or anxiety. We had bought a home and by now we had another child, my son Vinny. I had gone on to become an electrician, being that I took the electrical trade while in high school. From a small shop I ended up getting a job with the Federal Government working on an Air Force Base. Patty had graduated from college and was hired by the phone company. We were finally in a good financial situation and stable, we had new vehicles, a nice home, the children were happy and healthy and living the American Dream, until one day…

One evening, as Patty was making dinner, she began to call out my name in a hysterical state. I ran to the kitchen where I could see flames emerging from the cooking pan, almost touching the ceiling. I attempted to extinguish the fire by throwing flour on the flames, I covered the pan with a towel to no avail. Bryan and Vinny were both crying as they were scared as well. The smoke alarm activated with a loud high pitch noise. Out of reaction, I asked Patty to open the rear door by the kitchen leading to our patio. My idea was to grab the handle with a towel and take the pan right outside. Once

I saw Patty open the door, I took off with the pan, not realizing she had tripped and fell. As I was going out ,I tripped over her as she was getting up. The pan fell out of my hands, hitting the ground and a ball of flames came up from the pan under Patty's dress scorching her pantyhose to her legs. She began to scream in pain and horror.

I panicked and began to console her the best I could, constantly apologizing. The next thing you know, we were in the Emergency Room. Patty had sustained burns to her legs due to the pantyhose melting on her skin. We went home and I took care of her, changing her bandages every day. She would eventually heal and return to work. For now, all things were back to normal, or so I thought.

While at work and driving on a Military Base you must stop at any crosswalk if a pedestrian is waiting to cross. It could be frustrating at times, because if I failed to stop they would call in my vehicle number and my supervisor would have to give me a verbal warning. Now, what I was about to experience was another nightmare from hell. One morning while driving to a job site, I came up to one of these crosswalks. The people crossed over and all of a sudden, out of nowhere, I began to think that I ran over someone at the crosswalk. I found myself going back to the area where the pedestrian was waiting to cross. What am I thinking? I got to the point in which, once I got on base, I would tell the person I was working with that I was waiting on my eyeglasses and could not drive. I had no problems whatsoever with my eyesight but it allowed me not to drive. I made it through the day without having to drive around.

The bad part about it is I had to force myself to drive to work and back home. At times, when most were at home from work, I was still driving around the base, checking where I had driven to make sure I had not hit a pedestrian. I would tell myself, okay, just this one time. Nope, there I go again. Like a broken record the scenes would play in my head over and over. I envisioned a body full of blood on the roadway and me getting arrested for failing to stop and render aid. In all those times I never saw a body, there were never any police or ambulances at the locations. "Okay, no police or ambulance?" the monster would come in my mind and say,

"What if someone picked the hurt pedestrian up and gave him or her a ride to the hospital? I better park my vehicle and go check the road for blood. Whhhhhhhhhh... no blood, thank God! Wait a minute, was this the crosswalk or was it the other one?"

All this time, Patty and the kids were waiting for me to get home from work. I would have to force myself to leave the base. As I was driving home, my heart would race and if I saw an ambulance driving towards me, going the opposite direction, the one I had just come from, I began thinking they were on the way to tend to a person I may have hit. I would eventually make it home only to watch the news to make sure nobody was hit by a car similar to mine. This too would eventually take its toll on me. Patty thought I was obsessed with the news, not knowing what I was going through.

The OCD progressed. It went from the thought of running over someone with my vehicle to the thought of hurting people in general. I began to think that I may have physically hurt someone. One day at work, my friend Jack was on a ladder working on a light fixture, as I walked by him and passed, within a millisecond I imagined bumping into the ladder and he taking a bad fall. I turned my head and there he was, still on top of the ladder. Just to make sure I called out his name and made up some type of discussion with him to reassure myself he was okay. Later, I was in an office working alone when a pretty young lady was behind the desk. As I walked away I imagined that I had looked at her on an inappropriate manner and she had caught me. Thinking she might call my boss, I had to make sure everything was okay between her and I. I could not, however, come out and ask her, so I went back and acted as if I had forgotten something in the room, making sure she responded to my words, "Have a nice day", as I walked out. I asked myself, "What in the world is going on in my head now?"

Once again, I was back in the condition I was at seven years prior. This time even worse. In my tormented mind of OCD, I was running over pedestrians, accidently hurting people and returning to check over and over. I was out of control and going down fast. The problem became so serious that I could not back my vehicle out of our own driveway. And when I did make it out of the driveway, it was only a matter of time before I would encounter a jogger or someone on a bicycle, forcing me into another loop. If a piece of paper was on the roadway I panicked and slowed down, knowing what my eyes had seen, I would instantly imagine it was a small child on a bicycle or walking across the road, even perhaps a body that was on the roadway and I'd ran over. I would drive far from the curb side, away from morning walkers and avoided any bus-stops if possible.

My biggest fear was for Patty to ask me to take one of our children to school. The thought of all those children walking around would make me cringe. The OCD was so bad that not even a bug could fly by my headlights without me thinking it was a human body. I would have to return, not once, twice, three times, lose count and waste gas. All the time praying, asking God to help me. Please, Lord, take this away from me. Please!

I went to Patty with this problem. She began to sob telling me she did not know if she could handle going through this again. I told her to please bear with me, to not give up on me.

I begged her to not leave my side. I did, though, get to the point where I could not drive alone. If I drove it could only be with Patty as a passenger and I would tell her to keep an eye on the road for me. If she even turned her head to talk to the kids, I would get upset. I needed the reassurance that I did not run over someone. Patty was getting frustrated and could not take it anymore.

Once again, I was home-ridden and could not get out of the OCD world; I lived in fear. As I mentioned earlier, on top of the thoughts, I was dealing with anxiety attacks which would in turn become panic attacks. The thought of going to prison would frighten me to the point that I would rather not be driving around anyone so that I would not have to worry about those thoughts. I would not allow my person the opportunity to get into *any* situation. If I am not around anyone, if I am not driving, I am good. I was now a lost cause.

What to do? Who could help me? How could I go to a physiatrist and tell him or her what I was thinking? The first thing they would do is call the police thinking they had a serial killer in their office. Or would they admit me to a mental institution? I could not afford to go to a mental hospital.

Time was going by and I was once again missing work. I needed to find myself again. I was slowly drowning within my own mind. I needed someone to throw me a life jacket, quick.

The Phone Call

Sunday morning and we received a phone call from my wife's sister, Becky. Patty told me to go and get the paper from outside. Patty told me to look in the "San Antonio Life" section. I looked at the front page of this section and it read "The Phobia Clinic, patients dealing with panic and anxiety disorders and obsessive-compulsive disorder." I had no idea what those words meant.

Becky told Patty that she had read the section and it appeared that the patients had what I had. I opened the paper as if it were a gift, I couldn't believe what I was reading. These people had the same symptoms I was suffering with.

As Monday morning came, I called and made an appointment to see the doctor. Patty took the day off and we both went to the office. As we entered, there were other people sitting there. I looked at them and wondered if they felt like me. I was embarrassed to be there and was hoping that nobody would show up or work there that new me personally.

I was given a brochure to read. As I began to read it, I felt a giant weight lifted off my chest.

Finally, someone knows what I have. I could not wait to speak to the doctor.

The doctor would later come out and call my name. As he began to talk I could tell that he was of Middle Eastern descent. Very calm and collective, he asked me what my symptoms were. At first I was too scared to say, but I knew it was my chance to get some help. I was told that there was such a thing as Doctor and Client Privilege. What I tell him would remain between us. I opened up to him, letting him know all of my thoughts and the way I felt. When I would say I have these thoughts or those thoughts, I have this tightening on my chest, sweat, floating feeling, he would respond with, "Yes, that is normal". Normal? Who's the crazy one here? How could he say this is normal ? He would say, "You will be fine."

I kept talking and talking and it seemed as if he didn't want to hear anything more. I felt so confident that I wanted to tell him all. He finally gave me my prognosis: I was suffering from obsessive-compulsive disorder, in short known as OCD, which in turn would cause anxiety and panic attacks. I was informed that I had a biological problem due to the lack of a chemical in my brain that normally would allow me to get rid of thoughts. I was also informed that it was a condition that I inherited from either my father or mother. Now I was given two options to get cured: I could either take medication along with group therapy or I could be admitted to the hospital, which would be faster. My first question was, "Am I going to a mental hospital?" The doctor chuckled and smiled. He said, "No, you are not crazy. Remember you have a biological condition, not a mental condition". Good words of encouragement knowing now that yes, I did have a mental condition which was being caused by a medical condition.

I chose to go to the hospital. Patty, Bryan and Vinny were with me as I checked in. I was expecting to see people in straightjackets, talking to themselves. But instead, the people were acting normal. I met with the nursing staff and was led to a room. The nurse had no idea what I was talking about when I told her I had OCD. That night I was given my medication, Xanax and Prozac.

As I awoke, I went to the dining room for breakfast where I met some other patients. Almost all of them asked me what kind of drugs I was addicted too. When I told them I had OCD, they too had no idea what I was talking about. That was when I realized that I was in a Drug Rehabilitation Center.

The doctor came to visit me later that day and I asked him why I was in rehabilitation center for drug addicts. He explained to me that obsessive-compulsive disorder was a newly diagnosed condition and they still didn't have a facility to put such patients in. He wanted me to attend their group sessions as well.

I walked into the group one day and sat down. They all spoke of their battle with drugs and spoke about how I wanted drugs, well, the drug to cure my OCD. They could not understand what I was doing there. I didn't have much of a choice. I was also given word that I was to walk around with a female nurse for therapy. I now know what it was for, it was to get me to stop having thoughts and to realize that they were just that: thoughts.

Once my anxiety began to subside and my thoughts decreased, I was released with the suggestion to attend group therapy and one-on-one therapy. I still had a fear of driving.

6

Back home, I felt as if I had just landed on earth. Things seemed so much clearer in my head now, as if the windows had been cleaned. But I also felt like a new man and had missed out on some of my children's lives. Though I was only in the center for two weeks, it seemed like months. I knew that I was still not confident with my driving and had to attend not only driving therapy but group therapy as well.

My first day of group therapy was a surprising experience. As I entered the room I expected to see individuals in the bad condition I was in when I had not showered or shaven for days. There were a total of eight in the group which consisted of professionals, including a business owner, an older wealthy lady, and a young man who worked at a laboratory. The business owner began by sharing his story. He was at work, driving a large truck when he began to think he ran over some of the workers on the job site. Just like me, he got to the point where he could not drive anymore. Then there was this young man who worked in the laboratory and said he had a fear of getting germs so he constantly had to wash his hands. The elderly lady shared that she was suffering from panic attacks that started after she fell off one of her horses. It was then that I realized there were more phobias out there that I had not suffered with.

I worked on electricity and constantly got my hands dirty. As soon as it was time for lunch, there were times that I was so hungry I forgot to wash my hands. However, this young man's obsession was to keep his hands clean at all times, they termed him as a compulsive hand washer with the fear of germs.

As time went on and I attended several group sessions, I met several people with different fears which. The terminology commonly used amongst therapist is *phobias*, or as they would put it "boogy thoughts ". I met some with the phobia of driving and injuring someone, some could not even drive in fear of losing their own life, not hurting someone, like I did. Others suffered with the fear of crowds, speaking in public, not turning off their cigarette goodly enough, which could start a fire to the point that they would take the cigarette butt with them.

You see, what I learned was that there are several phobias that we all seem to have. However, without the medication and therapy needed to let go of that phobia, it can become compulsive and controlling. It goes back to not wanting to step on a crack on the sidewalk because that would bring bad luck if you don't go back and walk over it. I have even seen baseball players on television jump over the foul line or batters with repetitive rituals as they go up to bat; then there are those who have to keep their books and papers aligned on their desk; the one who has to touch a certain item a number of times. By the way, I had the touching case for a while. I would touch a light switch over and over until it felt right. If I left without that good feeling I would feel as if something bad was going to happen.

I found more about myself and my younger days, and how I had suffered with OCD all my life. It also is hereditary and I found out that my father, who was a smoker, had a metal coffee can with water in the patio where he would throw his cigarettes. I never told him anything, but I knew he was my genetic factor. My mother also told me that his father, who passed before I was born, suffered with anxiety to the point that he would eat standing up at times.

My first day of driving with Gina, the Therapist, we got into her vehicle and before leaving she lifted the rear-view mirror up to the point where I could not look back. She must have known that I would normally check and double check as I would pass by a pedestrian only to make sure the person was still walking on the sidewalk, etc. But after a while, I didn't even trust the mirror. I had to see it with my own eyes.

Before we left my hands began to sweat and my heart raced as I put the vehicle on drive. Passing by patients and others walking in the parking lot made me feel strange. I knew right then and there that I still had a long way to go until I could go back to work.

Gina told me to drive to the nearest mall. "A mall?" was the first thing that came to my mind. "Come on, lady, I can barely press the gas and you want me to go to the nearest mall?" But I told myself it was time to get this fear out of my system. I developed some courage and drive.

As we entered the mall I was fine because she was in the vehicle with me and I knew I had a witness just in case I "imagines" hitting someone with the vehicle. I went to park and Gina said, "No, don't park, just drop me off and take the car on the highway". She asked me to pick her up in thirty minutes. I was lost for words.

I did as she asked and began to drive. I did, though, make sure to drive on the inner lanes of the access road and get off and place myself in the inner lane once again. I didn't want to take the chance of having to see a pedestrian on the side of the road walking or broke down. I ended up going right back to the mall, parked and waited for the thirty minutes to come around.

After a few weeks of therapy, group sessions and taking my medication, like a flu bug, it just went away and I was back to normal. I would eventually make it back to work and through therapy I learned not to check or look back if I had a bad thought while driving. Within a few years I was driving 150 miles to Corpus Christi and back where I went to work on the Military Base.

One day, our team at work received information that there was going to be a huge lay off of employees. I was one to get laid off out of eight hundred and twenty government employees.

Normally I would have started to panic, but the medication made me deal with the situation; all I could think of was to not look back.

The Unbelievable

Believe it or not, I ended up applying for the Sheriff Department. I took the test and passed. I was called by a recruiter and told that I was to take a polygraph and a physiological exam. I thought for sure I was not going to get into the department due to my condition and the medications I was taking.

On the day I had a visit with the psychiatrist, he asked me to complete a questionnaire. I returned the form to him and he later spoke to me. I had to be honest, so when he read that I was taking Prozac and Xanax, he asked me why. I was straight forward and let him know that I had been diagnosed, in 1986, with obsessive-compulsive disorder, which caused me to have anxiety and panic attacks. There were still a lot of doctors, him included, that were not up to date with OCD, anxiety and panic attacks. Luckily for me, he knew my psychiatrist and told me that he would get back to me after speaking to him. I was called the next day and informed that I had been cleared to work for the Department.

I began my career in law enforcement working in the jail. There was a time that I was assigned to work in the Mental Health Unit. These inmates suffered with mental disorders of all types. A young inmate came up to me crying one day, he told me that the other inmates were saying he was going to prison. He stood in front of me rocking back and forth. I realized that having OCD was not that bad after all, considering the condition he was suffering with and the thoughts he could not seem to get over.

A few years went by and I went to the Patrol Division. While in the Patrol Division, all I did was drive around and at times had to drive fast on emergency calls, not even thinking of hurting someone on the road, but more concerned about getting in a wreck and damaging the car or myself. Amazing how one day I was literally handicapped in my home, living in terror, not even being able to back the vehicle out of our driveway, and then here I was strapped in a patrol car, going in circles through the neighborhoods with kids playing, people walking, and even going to schools to speak to students on Career Day.

I later took on the position of Crime Scene Investigator (C.S.I.). The fears that I had I would now see in real life as I worked the scene. I once made a vehicle pedestrian accident scene. The vehicle had sustained a lot of damage. I could not help but think about the damage I would have seen on my vehicle if I had ever accidently run over someone. I remembered getting home and looking at my vehicle up and down to see if there were any marks. While working these scenes I would get flashbacks of the horror I battled with in past days of my life.

The saddest scenes I made while working CSI were the suicides. Most all suicide victims leave a note behind. It was my job to take a photograph of the note and recover it as evidence. In reading some of the notes, I came across some victims who wrote, "I can't seem to get rid of these ugly thoughts", or merely suffered with depression or other psychological problem.

My heart would hurt for them because I knew exactly what they were going through, but they could no longer take it anymore. I never felt the urge to take my life, though I do remember asking God to take it for me. I didn't have the will and grew up being told that God does not like it when someone takes their own life and I could end up no telling where. I never shared my feelings with any of my fellow officers, I didn't want them to know I had OCD nor did I feel the necessity to tell them.

As years went by, I ended up getting promoted to the Homicide Division. I noticed that once I got on a case I could not let it go. I worked every angle possible and at times I would even take work home to study the files. Could it be a form of OCD that I still lived with? Is it possible that individuals who commit certain crimes have a form of OCD that doesn't let them control their thoughts? Not knowing right from wrong, they might not know how they have a chemical imbalance that makes them do what they do. That has and will always be a question that should be researched.

I was very successful with my cases and I can say that due to the drive and chemical imbalance that I have, I did not allow myself to let go of the case, almost as if having to drive back to check and see if I had run over someone. Now I am close to retirement and can say that though there are times I may have an intrusive thought or two, I know it is just that, simply a thought.

The brain is a strange thing, how can such a small mass in our head take over a human soul? It is unexplainable.

I suffered and overcame due to my strong wife and family who supported me through that dark cloud. I know I will forever have to take medication and it may have a long-term effect on my health. But, as in any illness or defect, we will all eventually have to take medication.

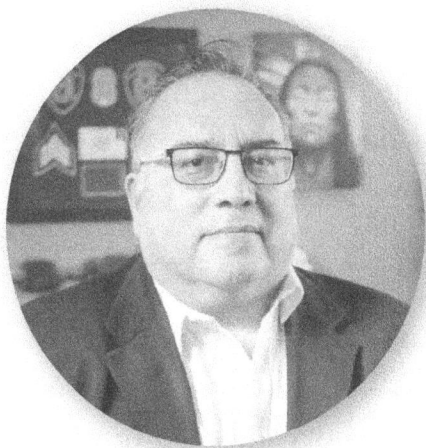

Adrian Ramirez is a retired Criminal Investigator who grew up with anxiety, panic attacks and what is now known as obsessive-compulsive disorder.

As a young boy, all he knew is that he felt afraid and scared. He did not want to go to school due to the unknown fear inside him. His parents could never understand why he was always afraid, but as he got older the symptoms subsided due to his involvement in clubs at school, such as student council, art club and athletics. It was in high school, as he participated in sports, where he felt at his best. At the age of 17 he graduated from high school and attended junior college. He later married at the age of 19 and had his first-born son.

Early in his marriage he sustained an eye injury, triggering the same anxiety and panic attacks he had as a child. The difference: this time he was a young adult, a new husband and young father living in a small apartment, trying to support his family and continue his studies, it all became overwhelming to young Adrian. Little did he know he was going to be facing the same demons once again, but now as an adult.

He spoke to several of his elders and finally reached out to his college counselor, who's explanation for his anxiety was that too many things were happening to him very fast and he was faced with so much new responsibility. Unfortunately, Adrian stopped going to school, could no longer work, and, worst of all, could no longer drive. His mind went spiraling out of control until he and his family moved from the small apartment to new surroundings. With the help of his wife, family members and prayers, he forced his way back into society where he could work and be there for his family.

For the next five years he was functional, but not to his full potential, struggling to survive the fear and anxiety day by day. It wasn't until a family member informed him of a local Phobia Clinic which appeared to be very familiar with what he was experiencing. He made an appointment with the clinic where both he and his wife were relieved to find out there was a name for his condition, obsessive-compulsive disorder, and that it was treatable.

Through months of therapy and medication, he became aware that it was actually intrusive thoughts that looped through his brain, creating the fear, anxiety and panic.

For something that Adrian thought he could never overcome; he was now able to control those intrusive thoughts. It was a long journey that no child or young adult should ever have to face.

Adrian has been commended and blessed as a wonderful husband, supportive father and an exceptional Law Enforcement Criminal Investigator. Understanding how treatment saved his life and that there may be others like him, Adrian advocates his experiences to those who have similar symptoms.

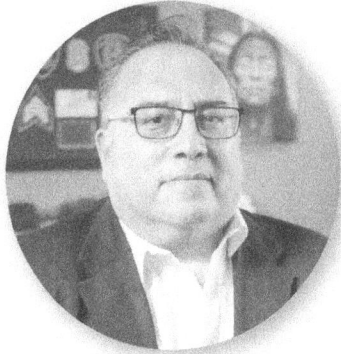

RETIRED CRIMINAL INVESTIGATOR

LET'S CONNECT

Get to know Adrian Ramirez.

Website:
www.Adrianramirez.info

Email:
aramirez3400@gmail.com

Facebook:
Adrian Ramirez

Instagram:
AuthorAdrianRamirez

www.ingramcontent.com/pod-product-compliance
Lightning Source LLC
LaVergne TN
LVHW021540080426
835509LV00019B/2753